A Concise Guide to Mastering the Medical School Interview

Dr. Regina Bailey, MD, JD

INTRODUCTION

In 2014, 49,474 people applied to medical school. Only 58% of first time applicants were admitted and 43% of the total applicant pool was admitted. The medical school application process is grueling, and the stakes are high, so you need to be as prepared as possible for your interview to gain a spot in medical school. The interview portion of the application process is extremely important, however, with a little planning and practice, this can be the easiest portion of the process. This book serves to be a guide to the medical school interview process and how to put your best foot forward and shine during your interview experience.

SCHEDULING THE INTERVIEW AND MAKING TRAVEL PLANS

Congratulations, you got an interview for medical school! So, what do you do now?

If you get an interview it means the admissions committee believes you can succeed academically in their school. At this point they want to get to know you and see if you are the type of person they want to train at their medical school.

Schedule Your Interview with the Coordinator

A coordinator from the school will contact you and give you available dates. Interview spots fill up fast, so schedule your interview date as soon as possible.

Make Travel Plans

If your interview is out of state, make travel arrangements as soon as possible. Try not to schedule arriving flights too late in the afternoon as flights frequently get delayed, and you want to be as rested as possible. Also, do not schedule your departing flights right after the scheduled conclusion of your interview. You do not want to be checking your watch and worrying that you are going to miss your flight, it can make the interviewers think you are not interested or preoccupied. You may also want some time after the interview to talk more with medical students or faculty that may stay around for further questions.

Check with the school to see if they offer housing with current medical students if that is something you would be interested in. If this is not something you are comfortable with, find a hotel to stay in. You can always get recommendations from the coordinator if you are unfamiliar with the area.

Some medical schools may have discounts with certain hotels already in place, so investigate that.

PREPARATION FOR THE INTERVIEW

In the months to days until your interview, there are very simple and key things you can do to prepare for your interview.

Know your personal statement, CV and any abstracts or articles that are on your CV in detail. It is a small world. Your interviewer may be involved in similar research, so you want to know the details of the project and what you contributed. Be prepared to explain any red flags, if any, in your application (grades, scores). Be prepared to explain gaps, if any, in your CV.

Research the school and prepare questions, but don't ask things that you can easily find on the school website. Research the faculty and prepare questions. You can ask them about the field of medicine they practice, how they decided to go into that field, their research, how they decided to do that type of research. Why did they pick that institution to work?

Research the different Types of interviews that you may encounter so that you are prepared for anything.

Traditional

In the traditional interview, you will meet one on one with someone from the medical school. Sometimes they will review your file ahead of time, sometimes they won't.

Panel

In the panel interview you will have multiple people are interviewing you at the same time.

Make eye contact with all the interviewers.

When one specific one is questioning you, make eye contact with them while they are talking, then continue while you are starting to answer the question, then make eye contact with the others as you are talking and finishing answering the question.

Blind

In the blind interview, the interviewer does not have access to your file. In this type of interview, you will likely get the "tell me about yourself" question as your first one, since they don't know anything about you. This type of interview is a good time to show your personality and enthusiasm for medicine without having to discuss grades, scores, etc.

MMI

MMI stands for "multiple mini interview."

This is a new interview technique for US medical school interviews. They are a series of short situations/scenarios that are used to assess your ethics, critical thinking, and communication skills. The purpose is not to test your knowledge in that area, but to see how you think though and react to the situation. It tests how you think on your feet. When you are in this situation remember that they are testing whether in their eyes, you are a good person, that makes good decisions, will make a good medical student and physician.

SAMPLE QUESTIONS

Practice, Practice, Practice…but don't be too rehearsed

These are sample questions that you may encounter in the medical school interview. After each question, I provide some tips for the question. These are not necessarily the answers you should give; I am just giving you information to start the thinking process.

GENERAL QUESTIONS

1. Tell me about yourself.

Tips: Most interviewers do not have the time or just do not want to review your application prior to the interview, so they will ask this question. Have a small story in your mind about yourself (Have a beginning, middle and end). For example, you can tell them where you are from, what are you currently doing in your life, and why you want to go to medical school?

2. Why do you want to be a doctor?

Tips: What motivated you to choose this profession? An interest in science? Mentor? Family member's illness? This is your time to discuss your passion and enthusiasm for medicine.

3. What type of medicine are you interested in?

Tips: Be flexible. You will see so many specialties in medical school; you want to be open and interested in everything. It is okay to have one field that interests you and discuss that, but make sure you have flexibility. You don't want to offend your interviewer that may be in a different field. Never say that you never want to do XYZ specialty or that you are not interested in XYZ specialty.

4. Why did you apply to this medical school?

Tips: Are you interested in specific research they do?

Do they have specific medical interests that you would like to pursue? International medicine, alternative medicine, public health?

Location; maybe you are looking for a change of scenery; want to practice medicine to the underserved in an urban area, practice medicine in a rural area?

5. Is this school your first choice, why?

Tips: You don't want to seem too eager, but you want to let them know that you are interested. You may want to say that it is early in the process and you are still evaluating all the schools to see which one is the best fit for you, if accepted.

6. What other schools are you applying?

Tips: They most likely don't have ill intents; they are just making conversation or are being nosy.

7. What would you if I gave you an acceptance letter today?

Tips: Be happy about that but also discuss needing to finish all your interviews before you decide. You want to be interested, but don't want to be "easy."

8. If you don't get accepted this year, what will you do?

Tips: Always answer that you will reapply and have some back-up plan as to what you will do in the year you are waiting to reapply (research, post-baccalaureate, work). Medicine is a very grueling profession; you want to show that you can handle rejection and continue towards your goals.

9. What exposure to medicine have you had?

Tips: If you don't have any exposure, get some now. Volunteer in a hospital or clinic. Find a mentor to shadow.

10. We have a lot of qualified applicants, why should we choose you?

Tips: Discuss your strengths, what you are good at, what you are proud of. Try to tie your interests to the school (making a connection). "I'm interested in this…. And you do this….."

11. If interviewing in a state you don't live in, be prepared to answer: "Why do you want to move to XYZ."

Tips: It's good to have connection to the area, or at least a reason why you want to live there (change in climate, new environment, desire to practice medicine in an underserved community).

12. If you get multiple acceptances, how will you decide?

Tips: Evaluate all the schools and determine which the best fit is; consider cost, location, etc.

13. What do you think is the biggest challenge in medicine today?

Tips: Access, Cost, Insurance, etc. Tons of areas you can talk about. Talk about an area that you are interested in or are knowledgeable about.

14. What do you think will be your biggest challenge in medical school and what will you do to work on it?

Tips: Think about what challenges you expect and how you will you will work on it.

15. What scares you about medical school?

Tips: Be honest. Most people have some fear of medicine. The hours of studying, gross anatomy lab, less time for hobbies. But discuss that you have thought though the rigors of medicine and have thought of ways to combat these fears and be prepared.

Another subject you can discuss is the politics and business of medicine and interfering with you providing care to your patients.

16. What scares you about medicine?

Tips: See #15

17. What was your favorite class in college (science and non-science) and why?

Tips: Probably more of a getting to know you type question but be prepared for it.

18. What things do you think you have to change or give up when you become a doctor?

Tips:

You may not necessary have to give up things, but you can discuss that you may have to be more flexible, adjust your lifestyle; e.g., manage time wisely, be on a budget while in medical school.

ETHICAL QUESTIONS

(these are also the types of scenarios that you may see in the MMI type of interview).

19. Impairment. What would you do if you found out that one of your fellow students had a substance abuse problem?

Tips: Talk to them, see if you can help them find some help.

20. Cheating. What would you do if you found out that one of your fellow students had a copy of the next anatomy exam and asked if you wanted to see it?

Tips: It would be tempting to look at the exam, but you sacrificed too much to get into medical to put that into jeopardy by cheating.

Would you report it? Consider reporting anonymously.

21. Right to die/euthanasia

Tips: Know the basics about it and the laws in your state. If you are for it, be prepared to explain why. If you are against it, be prepared to explain why.

22. Consent. A patient refuses a lifesaving treatment based on their religious beliefs, what would you do?

Tips: If they have the capacity to make consent, they have the right to refuse care. You as the physician also must respect their beliefs. You should discuss the seriousness of it with the patient, the risk of death if they do not have the treatment. Give the patient the information, but ultimately you must respect their wishes. You may want to discuss how this makes you feel and how you would personally deal with it.

23. How would you tell a patient that they have HIV, terminal cancer, etc.

Tips: Take them to a private area, discuss with them the diagnosis. Allow them to process it. Allow time for questions, feelings, etc.

24.If you were driving, saw an accident on the street, would you stop and help?

Tips: Offer to help up to your level of training (only do CPR if you are CPR trained). Would it be safe to stop and help, or would you put others in danger?

25. If you are on an airplane and someone is ill, would you volunteer to help?

Tips: Offer to help up to your level of training (only do CPR if you are CPR trained) if you felt you could be of assistance and would like to help. If you are not comfortable helping, you can discuss that you don't have the training yet, but after finishing medical school you may be better served to help in such an emergency.

AFORDABLE CARE ACT and OTHER POTENTIAL HEALTH INSURANCE QUESTIONS

26. health care a right or a privilege?

Tips: Think about why or why not.

27. What do you think about the Affordable Care Act? What do you think needs to be done to make it better?

Tips: Think about what the good features about the Affordable Care Act are, for example, maybe because of the law you are now covered under your parent's insurance, and had that not been in place, you may not have been able to afford health insurance. You could discuss the patients that could not get health insurance because of preexisting conditions, but now are covered and can get treatment for those illnesses. Things that you could suggest adding, providing more access to health care providers by increasing the funding and size of residency programs, build more medical schools, etc. Again, these are not the answers that you should give; I am just giving you things to start the thinking process.

28.What is the difference between Medicare and Medicaid?

Tips: Some interviewers may choose to quiz you about the basics of health insurance to see if you know the basics about the field you are going into.

Medicare is a health insurance program run by the federal government. It covers people that are 65 years old and older and younger people with End-Stage Renal Disease and are on dialysis.

Medicaid is a health insurance funded and run by both the federal and state governments and helps people with health care costs if they have a lower income. In most states it will also cover women who have no health insurance when they become pregnant and some states have Medicaid programs that cover children in families with lower incomes.

It may be a good idea to review your state's Medicaid program.

29.What is the difference between an HMO and a PPO?

Tips:

HMO stands for Health Maintenance Organization. It gives the individual access to doctors and hospitals with in its network. These providers have agreed to provide lower rates for people in the HMO. Care is only covered if you see a provider within that network. Your primary care physician must refer you to a specialist if they think you need it.

PPO stands for Preferred Provider Organization. A PPO has a network but is less restrictive the HMO. It will pay for visits to out of network providers, but it will likely be a lower rate of coverage than your in-network provider. You do not need to see your primary care doctor to get a referral for a specialist, you can just pick one, make an appointment and go. Because of this flexibility, PPO premiums are higher than

HMO premiums.

ACCESS TO HEALTH CARE

30.What is a solution to the shortage of primary care physicians?

Tips: Consider discussing increase the number of medical schools, residency spots, and funding for these programs. Provide more loan forgiveness or repayment for physicians that specialize in primary care.

31. What should we do about the cost of healthcare in the United States?

Tips: Overuse of the system? Over testing? Defensive medicine?

PHYSICIAN LIFE

32. Is there anything that scares you about being a physician?

Tips: Be honest, are you scared of anything? Maybe going to the anatomy lab for the first time. Scrubbing into your first surgery. Maybe the lifestyle scares you. Discuss that the fears aren't stopping you from achieving your goals.

33. Where do you see yourself in 15 years?

Tips: Academic, Private Practice, Administration. Start a family. It's okay to say you don't know, but at least think generally what you see yourself doing, even if it is a big dream. Run your own hospital.

34. What are you most proud of?

Tips: This is a time to brag about yourself (without being cocky).

35. What has been the greatest obstacle in your life?

Tips: This is a good time to discuss something that you had difficulty with but worked on and improved.

36. What do you think about alternative medicine?

Tips: Don't discount it. You need to be open to your patient's beliefs. Discuss how you may be able to incorporate it into traditional medicine. For example, discuss with your patient continuing to take their blood pressure medication, but it is also okay for them to try acupuncture, vitamins, etc.

37. How do you think the internet has changed the practice of medicine?

Tips: People get a tremendous amount of information on the internet, I call it Dr. Google. You must be able to discuss with your patient information they find on the internet and why it may or may not be applicable to them. People also rate doctors on the internet. What are your feelings about that?

38. Would you accept a Facebook friend request from a patient?

Tips: Think about the ethics of that, the doctor-patient relationship, professionalism, boundaries, etc.

39.What do you think of PA's and NP's doing work that was once done only by doctors? Do you feel like they are taking your job?

Tips: Remember, you need to be a team player. Access to medicine is already a huge problem and will only get worse has more people will be eligible for health insurance.

PA's and NP's, under the guidance of physicians, can greatly help improve access to medicine.

PERSONALITY/SOCIAL QUESTIONS

40. If I talked to your friends about you, what would they say about you?

41. What are your positive qualities?

42.What are your strengths?

43. What are your negative qualities?

Pick a negative quality that you have worked on and discuss how you have improved it. They are looking to see if you can be aware of your limitations, that you are willing to improve those limitations.

44.What are your weaknesses? Same as #43

45. Are you a leader or follower?

Depends on the situation, sometimes I am the leader, other times, someone is more qualified for the position and because I am a team player, I am a follower.

46. How do you work in team situations?

You must be able to work in teams in medicine. Sometimes you will need to take the lead, other times others will lead, but you must be able to get along and be a productive member of the team.

47. What is a good physician?

Caring, compassionate, efficient, team player, good communicator, etc.

48. What qualities about you will make you a good physician?

Caring, compassionate, efficient, team player, good communicator, etc.

49. How do you deal with stress?

Hobbies go for a walk, family time, sports.

Medical school is very stressful, and medicine is a very stressful career, they want to know how you are going to be able to deal with the stress.

50. Tell me something funny?

Have a clean joke ready or a funny story about yourself.

51. Who is your hero?

52. What are your hobbies? Do you plan to continue your hobbies in medical school?

Medical schools want well rounded, sociable people. There are things about your hobbies that can make you a good doctor. It is also a good way to de-stress. Medicine is a stressful career and they want to know that you have a life outside of medicine.

53. Do you do any volunteer work?

54. What do you do for fun?

55. What was the last movie you saw?

56. What is the last non-medical, non-scientific book you have read for pleasure?

57. What is a goal you had that you reach and how did you reach it?

58. Have you ever failed at something and how did you deal with it?

59. If you could change anything about your personality what would you change?

Be proud of yourself, don't change anything.

60. If you could do your life over again, what would you do differently this time?

61. Is there anything else you would like to add?

This is a time to talk about anything you didn't get to that you would like the interviewer to know about.

INTERVIEW THE INTERVIEWER

Often at the end of the interview, interviewers will ask you if you have any questions. Remember that you are interviewing the school also. You need to find out if this medical school is a good fit for you. Can you see yourself there for four years?

Some medical schools will let you know ahead of time who will be interviewing you (may be days ahead or the morning of your interview). If you have this information, try to do a little research about your interviewer. Read about them on the school's website. Have questions about their field of medicine. If they do research, have questions about their research. If they have a hobby, ask them about that. You want to show interests in the interviewer (without being stalker-ish) that will help to make a connection. Interviews are all about making a positive connection with your interviewer.

SAMPLE QUESTIONS TO ASK THE INTERVIEWER

1. What is their typical day like?

2. How did they decide to go in that field?

3. Where did they go to medical school?

4. Do they do research, what type?

5. How is living in XYZ city?

6. USMLE Passage rates

7. Has the school been on probation or had any accreditation issues?

8. What is their opinion about the school?

9. Research opportunities?

QUESTIONS TO ASK THE STUDENTS

You should have some time allocated to talk to current medical students. Here are a few suggestions of questions you may want to ask.

1. What is their opinion about the school?

2. Are they happy there?

3. Is there anything they would change about the school?

4. What attracted them to the school?

5. Ask about questions you may have about their clinical and non-clinical curriculum.

6. Ask if there are any clinical opportunities in your non-clinical years.

7. Do they get elective time?

8. Are there any note taking services? Who runs it?

9. Volunteer opportunities?

10. Research opportunities?

11. What is the grading system?

12. Student organizations and activities?

13. What do they think of the study space?

14. How do they evaluate their professors?

15. Are there any counseling services?

16. Is there a mentor program?

17. Are there any diversity programs?

18. What hospitals available for clinical rotations? How far are they from the medical school? Do you need a car to get there?

19. Housing and transportation

INAPPROPRIATE QUESTIONS

Prepare for inappropriate questions that you may encounter. Some interviewers may ask racist or sexist questions, because they either want to see how you react or they are just flat out inappropriate.

This is an example of a question I had in a medical school interview. "Why should we give you the spot if you are just going to stop practicing medicine to have children, aren't we wasting that spot?" I answered that many women have successfully managed a medical career and a family, that I didn't plan to stop practicing medicine if I did decide to have a family and that women are great multi-taskers and if anyone can do both, we can.

Think about how you will react and respond to any inappropriate questions.

ATTIRE

The way you physically present yourself at your interview may affect the interviewer's decision. There is not much you can control in the interview process, but this one area that you control, and you can address with a fool proof plan.

Dress as professionally as possible. Someone once gave me the advice that you always want to dress one level above the job you are applying for (meaning, if applying for medical school, dress as you expect someone would in applying for a residency or physician spot). This is advice that I still use today for my job interviews.

Invest in at least 2 good interview suits. I recommend going with solid colors (Black, Navy Blue, or Grey). Make sure your suit is not too big or too small.

For women, if you wear a skirt, make sure your skirt is not too short and please wear pantyhose. Make sure you are not showing cleavage. I recommend a white or cream-colored blouse for under your suit.

For men, wear a full suit (not just shirt and tie). Your tie should be solid color or have a print that is not too busy.

Wear comfortable shoes. During your interview you are likely to get an extended tour of the medical school facilities and hospitals. If your heels are too high you will be very uncomfortable and that is something you do not want to worry about on your interview day. Stick with a chunky low heel or flat shoes. I would advise you to go with a solid color for shoes as well. Your shoes should be closed toe. For men I recommend dark business shoes, with matching socks.

Keep your hair neat, clean and have it pulled back off your face if you have long hair. Again, you don't want to have to deal with constantly fixing your hair that day. Beards, mustaches should be neatly trimmed.

Carry a nice portfolio and/or briefcase. If you carry a purse, keep it simple.

Do not wear a lot of perfume or cologne and please keep your make-up simple. Do not wear a lot of accessories, keep that simple as well. A nice pair of pearl earrings and necklace is always fool proof.

Overall, you want to be dressed professionally. You do not want to have any part of your appearance to distract from your interview. You want eyes focused on your face, what you are saying and nothing else. If you have a distracting outfit, appearance, etc, it will take the attention away from what you are saying and may hurt your interview chances. I am not saying don't be yourself, but the interview is not the time for you to show everything you have. Remember what your goal is, to become a doctor. Dressing appropriately and professionally is one easy step that you can control to get to your goal.

INTERVIEW DAY TIPS

What to do the day before your interview:

- If you are flying, try to take your suitcase (or at least your suit) on board with you. The last thing you need is getting your luggage lost and having to interview in a T-shirt and shorts. Pack an extra suit just in case something happens (like spill coffee on yourself the morning before your interview).

- If the school is having a social activity the night before, have fun, but be aware that your behavior will be observed. Do not drink too much alcohol.

- Visit the campus (take a test drive)

• Get a good night sleep. If you are traveling, try to arrive early enough to get settled, look around, do something fun or rest.

What to do the day of your interview:

• Arrive early.

• Bring over the counter medicine with you just in case you have a headache or get sick (ibuprofen, acetaminophen, cold medicine, etc).

• Bring an extra pair of pantyhose in case you get a run in the one you are wearing.

• Check your teeth and breath after the lunch

• Make good eye contact

• Give a firm hand shake

• Try to not talk too fast.

- Do not be negative or put down other institutions (even if they are rivals)

- When you feel nervous, remember that although these are physicians with many more years of experience than yourself and may have a say in your fate in the admission process, they are just real people. We go to the bathroom, eat, pay taxes and die, just like everyone else.

What to do after your interview:

- Thank your interviewer for their time; tell them it was nice talking to them. Ask the coordinator when decisions are made.

- Breathe, relax and do something fun. Treat yourself.

- Do not say anything negative on social media. This is a rule for the whole application process.

Remove anything that may be considered inappropriate from your social media accounts. Some schools look at social media accounts and you don't want that to be the reason you aren't given a spot.

• Send a thank you note to your interviewer. In your note you should reiterate why you are interested in attending that school, why you would be a good candidate there. Keep it short and sweet. Remember that anything you send most likely will end up in your admissions file, so keep it professional.

CONCULSION

In a nutshell, practice interviewing, make good travel plans and make them early, dress professionally, act professionally, relax and breathe. You can do this. Congratulations and good luck

ABOUT THE AUTHOR

Dr. Regina Bailey is an Emergency Medicine Physician, Lawyer, Fitness Expert, Former NFL Cheerleader, Beauty Queen, Best Selling Author, and Motivational Speaker.

Dr. Regina received a BA in Molecular Biology from Hampton University, JD from Georgetown University, MD from the George Washington University School of Medicine, and Masters in Health Law from the University of Houston Law Center.

Prior to attending law school, she did biomedical research at Yale University, Stanford University and the National Institutes of Health. Prior to attending Medical School, she was a patent attorney in Washington, DC where she fought for the rights of generic drug companies to get their lower cost drugs on the market.

She completed an Internship in General Surgery at University of Texas Health Science Center at Houston and completed Emergency Medicine Residency at the Baylor College of Medicine.

She has published books and articles in the health law, medical, biotechnology and Emergency Medicine fields. She speaks on the above topics, as well as medical school admission tips, fitness, surviving sexual assault, and choice motherhood. She has appeared on TLC, Discovery Life Channel, CNN, and the E! Channel. She has been published in the New York Times, US News, Medscape, Huffington Post and Ebony Magazine. During her free time, Dr. Regina she competes (and wins) pageants and fitness competitions.

Dr. Regina is CEO of "Fit and Fine in No Time" a company that provides, nutritional supplements, meal replacement shakes and weight loss products all formulated by herself.